Ketogenic Diet

Types of Keto Diet and Precautions While You Lose Weight

Ben Harewood

© 2016

TABLE OF CONTENTS

INTRODUCTION

A brief Intro to Ketogenic Diet

A Ketogenic diet consists of high amount of fats and low amount of fats. Numerous studies have shown the health benefits of Ketogenic diet. This diet is also proven to reduce the symptoms of grave diseases such as cancer, diabetes, Alzheimer's disease, and epilepsy. Often called as Keto, this diet is similar to regular low-carb and Atkins diets. In this nutritional regime, you care supposed to drastically reduce your intake of carbohydrates and consume large amount of fat in its place. When you cut down on eating carbs, your body enters a metabolic state known as ketosis.

In the state of ketosis, your body burns fats to produce energy very efficiently. It also transforms fats into the ketones in your liver to supply energy to your brain. You might witness massive reduction in you levels of insulin and blood sugar, which provides many benefits with increased amount of ketones.

Normally, our body uses carbohydrates as fuel to provide energy to the body. However, when we stop consuming carbs or consume negligible amount of it, our body has to adapt itself to use another source to create energy. Along with South Beach Diet and Atkins diet, people who have interest in low carbohydrate method of dieting are likely looking at the Ketogenic diet. If you want to lose weight quickly or maintain your blood sugar level, you need to eat fat for losing fat. For this purpose, you need to bring the level of carbs in your body to 50 grams a day or less. Some dieticians will even advise you to consume maximum 30 grams of carbohydrates a day. However, it depends on person-to-person what amount of carbohydrates suit them to be in the state of ketosis.

How to set up the Ketogenic diet

To set up the Ketogenic diet, you have to take the lean body mass of your body. Lean Body Mass refers to that composition of your body, which is calculated if you subtract your weight of body fat from the weight of total body. It means that total body weight refers to body fat plus lean body mass.

You can write it in an equation as follows:

'LBM is equal to BW – BF'

Once you calculate your lean body mass, multiply the LBM by one. You will get the amount of proteins (in grams) you need to eat in a day. Now, multiply this number by 4 (because there are four calories in one gram protein) to obtain the total number of calories that you will get from protein.

Your remaining requirement of nutrients will be received from fat calories. That is why; there is no requirement to estimate the grams of carbohydrates specifically since you will automatically eat 30-50 grams of carbs every day when you eat green vegetables. In addition, there are incidental carbohydrates that are included in the source of protein and fats.

To estimate the grams of fat you need, you can subtract the protein calories from the number of calories required to maintain the weight of your body (which is 14-16 calories for each pound of your body weight). Divide the resulting number by 9 (which is the number of calories in one-gram fat). The final number is the total amount in grams of fats you are required to consume each day.

To calculate the number of meals you wish to eat daily, divide the resulting number by it. This will give you the layout of your basic diet. You must make sure that you consume plenty of leafy green vegetables to have proper amount of vitamin and antioxidant protection.

Carb load for weekends

After the entire week of following Ketogenic diet, everyone needs some relaxation from the strict regime. You can have a weekend period of carb load, which is usually great fun for most people. During this phase, you can eat huge amounts of food that contain carbs such as cereal, bagels, candy, pasta, and rice chips.

Since you would not eat much fat during this phase, there are lesser chances that carbohydrates will be converted into fat since your body will use these carbs to full up the store of muscle glycogen once again. You can choose a weekend period such as Friday night to Saturday night to begin the carb up phase. Since you do not have to go to work on weekends, it becomes easy to follow the regime and enjoy it as well. You do not have to be too much concerned about the fat loss. You can simply use the Ketogenic diet to maintain the level of blood sugar. You can eat almost any kind of carbohydrate containing foods during this phase. Do not worry too much about gaining body fat. If you are still concerned, you need to calculate the basics again.

You must try to keep the protein at one gram in each pound of your body weight. Then, consume 10-12 grams carbs for each kilogram of your body weight. Consume these carbohydrates (normally in liquid form in the first bit) right after you are back from the gym on Friday evening. This is the time when the body is prepared and it can uptake carbohydrates to provide you the maximum benefits.

CHAPTER 1

Types of Ketogenic diet

Ketogenic diet is not just consuming less carbs and a lot of fat. You have to be extra careful about the kind of food you eat according to the various branches of Ketogenic diet. Broadly, Ketogenic diet can be classified as follows:

- Targeted Ketogenic Diet or (TKD
- Cyclical Ketogenic Diet or (CKD)
- Standard Ketogenic Diet or (SKD)
- Restricted Ketogenic Diet (Therapeutic Uses)

You cannot strictly implement any of these diets. Every person is distinct regarding his or her needs of nutrition. You must experiment with different plans to find out what suits you the best. Some of you may find the 15-day Cyclical Ketogenic Diet best for their body, while the others may prefer to have a carb load on a weekly basis. It gives you more sovereignty to choose the finest option for you.

If you exercise intensely, you can make carbohydrates coexist with the process of ketosis. In case you do not intend to force your body for maximum physical development or defeat your performance plateau, you must not go too far with the consumption of carbohydrates.

Which diet you should choose from the given alternatives

If you are asking yourself this question, you just need the basic Standard Ketogenic Diet. TKD and CKD are meant for those who are well aware of their limits or who cannot break through or achieve their ceiling without consuming carbs. TKD and CKD are mostly used in the exercises of very high intensity and they must never be utilized as a pretext to consume anything sweet before your workout.

If you are not exercising too hard, you do not have to go through TKD and CKD. These two types of Ketogenic diets are meant only for those people who test the limits of their body and do not eat carbs to satisfy their cravings.

Which type of Ketogenic diet gives the best results?

One cannot give a straightforward answer for this question since the diet is always based on your intake of calories. If you keep your calorie intake constant, any of these diets may give similar results.

Standard Ketogenic Diet

SKD is the widespread type of Ketogenic diet because of its thumb rule; you just need to eat minimum amount of carbohydrates every day. If you are aware of the induction stage of Atkins diet, you will find it similar to it. It needs approximately 20-25 grams net carbohydrates per day. However, this amount may change according to an individual's needs. For those who do not want to go into the depths of Ketogenic diet shall adopt Standard Ketogenic Diet.

SKD consists of low carbohydrates, high fats, and moderate proteins. You can only consume carbs from fibrous vegetables and completely avoid milk, starch, or fruits. You are also encouraged to consume cheese and fatty parts of meat, cooked in oils and butter. You have to follow the same diet throughout the week. While you can follow this diet round the week, you can work out as you do simultaneously.

Who can adopt Standard Ketogenic Diet?

If you engage in high intensity workouts, you must not adopt the Standard Ketogenic Diet. This diet is meant for regular folks who do not work out much since there is not much consumption of regular carbs. It is a good diet for those who conduct a sedentary way of life with little aerobics or no exercise at all. It can be a great alternative for those who are heavily overweight or find the idea of exercising very uncomfortable. You can start losing fat with SKD and help resist the temptation for carbohydrates and control your hunger pangs. Once your weight reaches your desired level, you can include more carbs in your diet and you can exercise without much pain.

Advantages and disadvantages of Standard Ketogenic Diet

Apart from the gains of Ketogenic diet such as feeling full after meals, decreased hunger, there are several advantages and disadvantages of Standard Ketogenic Diet.

Advantages

- Regulates cravings for carbohydrates
- Controls hunger pangs
- You can lose weight without exercising

Disadvantages

- Not much variety of food is there because of restriction on carbohydrates
- It becomes difficult to maintain the diet without disrupting it sometimes by consuming carbs
- Hormones responsible for fat loss (ghrellin, leptin) are required to be reset to maintain the process of weight loss. They cannot be reset without eating higher carbs on a few occasions.
- You can sustain only low power exercises such as slow cycling and walking.

Targeted Ketogenic diet

Targeted Ketogenic diet is a more traditional approach to this plan. According to this regime, you are required to eat carbohydrates about an hour or a half before you go for workout. Since you are going to exercise after a while, you must consume carbohydrates that can be easily digested. Such carbohydrates have high Glycemic Index so that your stomach does not get upset when you consume them. You must avoid foodstuff that contains high amount of fructose. You can rather go for foods based on glucose. Fructose replenishes glycogen in liver, in place of glycogen in muscles, which you have to avoid in Ketogenic diet.

It implies that the carbohydrates that are eaten prior to exercising are utilized effectively. They are entirely burnt and do not interrupt with ketosis for a long period. Ideally, you can consume 30-50 grams of net carbohydrates an hour before workout. After you return home, your diet must consist of low fats and high proteins. Although fat is healthy for people following Ketogenic diet in general, but if you consume too much of it after workout, it may hamper absorption of nutrients and recovery of muscles. That is why; you need to avoid eating high fat foodstuff after exercise.

The older studies used to state that people should consume high carbohydrate- food if they engage in extremely intense exercises. However, recent studies outdate this approach.

How MCTs can boost your working

It is not necessary that you have to eat carbohydrates before workout, if your body does not allow. In reality, some people may completely disrupt their routine by consuming carbs like that. It may impair their performance in adaptation for Ketogenic diet. What works for one person may not work for the others. Few people may perform better with TKD or by consuming carbohydrates prior to workout, particularly if they are engaged in vigorous exercising that needs explosive actions. If you do not want to do it, you can try and watch how your body performs without carbohydrates intake. Your body takes at least a month to get adapted to Ketogenic. During this period, you must take your workouts easily.

If you have an active lifestyle, but you want to keep away from carbohydrates, you can start consuming coconut oil in place of regular vegetable oils. Coconut oil is the finest source of Medium Chain Triglycerides or MCT, which can be digested without much effort by the body. They are not stored in your body; therefore, they can be immediately used for creating energy. Research proves that MCTs are great fat burners because of their thermogenic properties.

In place of pre-exercise carbohydrates, you can consume snacks made of coconut oils. You will hardly notice any difference whether you consume carbohydrates or not. After your body adapts to Ketogenic diet, it begins using fat and ketones as fuel and does not require any carbohydrates.

Simply put, TKD or Targeted Ketogenic Diet is just like common Ketogenic diet, with an exception of consuming carbohydrates prior to your regime of workouts. It means that whenever you plan to exercise during the week, you need to consume carbohydrates. If you aim to lose fat through Keto, you need to ensure that you include additional calories from your carbs when you total them. At last, you just need to remember that you eat fewer fats when you exercise.

Advantages of TKD or Targeted Ketogenic Diet

You can call TKD as a mid-way between CKD and SKD, or Cyclical Ketogenic Diet and Standard Ketogenic Diet. It implies that you can still work out heavily, but you need stay out of the process of ketosis for a long time period.

In general, TKD is able to fulfill the needs of most people who wish to exercise and still be in ketosis. Even though TKD is good enough for most people, it is not as useful as CKD. Medium Chain Triglycerides

Targeted Ketogenic Diet is particularly useful for the beginners, those who practice training of intermediate strength or those cannot implement CKD or Cyclical Ketogenic Diet because of health issues. By now, no studies have presented the restraints of weight training supported on lower consumption of blood glucose. However, there are a few studies, which place carbohydrates before strength training and resistance, but they could not prove any enhancement in performance in the long term. There are many supporters of TKD, who report improvement in strength and endurance in high intensity atmosphere when they consume carbohydrates prior to workouts.

Individuals engaged in anaerobic workout on the Standard Ketogenic Diet particularly give an account of improved performance when they consume moderate-carb diet before workout. The only issue with SKD is that it can limit you to low intensity workouts because of limited muscle glycogen and glucose.

If you engage in high intensity workouts, you must experiment with various levels of carbohydrates during your period of training. Even though your performance increases in TKD or Targeted Ketogenic Diet, it is not your primary aim. The basic goal here is to maintain the level of glycogen in your body so that you can prepare your body for the next session of workout.

Sources of carbohydrates in Targeted Ketogenic Diet

Most individuals that test with Targeted Ketogenic Diet find out that 30-50 grams of carbohydrates give best results, if consumed half an hour before the workout. The majority of people suggest simple eating of easily digestible carbohydrates like foods containing high glycemic levels or liquids for faster absorption in the body. You can also eat white bread, sweet tarts, or candy bars.

The finest sources of carbohydrates for TKD are glucose and dextrose, which can be consumed from hard candies, gummy bears, Gatorade, or Powerade. There are some people who take organic maple syrup before workout and claim good results.

Some people claim that their body quits ketosis quickly for a while after they work out because of increased level of insulin. Since blood glucose gets absorbed in the muscles, the level of insulin drops and ketosis must start again. If you are concerned about this fact, you can practice cardio exercises with low intensity to help lower the level of insulin and augment free fatty acids in blood.

Carbohydrates after workout are more noticeable since the level of insulin is more elevated. That is why; it is strongly suggested that you start with consuming carbohydrates only before workouts, and add them after exercising only if you feel they are necessary.

Cyclical Ketogenic Diet

The first thing you must know about Cyclical Ketogenic diet is that this diet plan is not meant for everyone. Even if you are vigorously active, you do not have to do carb backloading or carb cycling. It totally depends on the kind of exercise you do and other preferences.

In Cyclical Ketogenic Diet, you are required to alternate the days of Ketogenic dieting and the days of high carbohydrates consumption. The latter is also called carb-loading. Ideally, the phase of carb-loading is 24-48 hours long. During the normal days, you can consume 50 grams of carbohydrates per day, and during the carb-loading days, you can consume 500-600 grams of carbohydrates. Athletes and bodybuilders use CKD plan to exploit fat loss while creating lean mass. That is why; this diet is not meant for common folks.

The bodybuilders have a common misconception about CKD that ketosis indicates breakdown of proteins. However, this is absolutely wrong and the truth is exact opposite this myth. In CKD, the body adapts to ketosis and minimum muscle tissues. When your body is fed with protein and fat, it uses body fat and dietary fat for energy and protein goes towards building muscles.

Cyclical Ketogenic Diet and Targeted Ketogenic Diet are much advanced levels of Ketogenic diet for most people and hence they should be adopted by only highly active people. You cannot use CKD and TKD for consuming cheat meals with high amount of carbohydrates every week.

In place of consuming small portions of carbohydrates before and after your exercise, the CKD makes you eat high amounts of carbohydrates two complete days in a week to entirely replenish the stores of muscle glycogen. You have to be a professional athlete to perform a successful Cyclical Ketogenic Diet. You need to completely deplete the stores of glycogen to have a successful Cyclical Ketogenic Diet.

CKD is definitely meant to build your muscles in the shortest time possible, but the flipside is that you might build some fat in your body. It is easy to gain fat, indulge in overeating, and have severe depletion workouts. If you are a beginner for CKD, you must start it under the guidance of a professional, or you can simply undertake Targeted Ketogenic Diet or Standard Ketogenic Diet.

The typical format for CKD is following the Ketogenic diet for 5-6 days and eating high- carb foods for 1-2 days. However, there are people who experiment with the cycle of 2 weeks, where they practice Ketogenic diet for 10-12 days and 3-4 days of carbohydrates eating. This splitting of Cyclical Ketogenic Diet also give good results but it does not fit in the schedule for everyone.

The main aim here is to come out of the phase of ketosis for the time being to replenish muscle glycogen to sustain performance of training in the coming cycle. If you plan to adopt Ketogenic diet for treating your health issues such as hypertension or hyperinsulinemia, Cyclical Ketogenic Diet may not be suitable for you. This is because sudden consumption of carbohydrates may trigger symptoms of your health conditions, which are specifically treated by consuming negligible carbohydrates.

CKD aims at completely depleting the muscle glycogen; you need a proper schedule of workouts to have the best results. A good example of workout can be:

A complete body split on Monday and Tuesday. You can do abs and legs on Monday, and do arms, chest, and back on Tuesday.

You can do work out of extreme rep depletion for the entire body on Friday.

The amount of workout to deplete the level of glycogen in your body depends on the carbohydrates amount you had in the carb-loading phase. If you used heavy weight, low rep; then only 2-3 sets may be required. On the other hand, if you used moderate weights, high rep, you might need to perform 5-6 sets.

How you can do Cyclical Ketogenic Diet

The phase of consuming low carbohydrates is similar to that of Standard Ketogenic Diet. You can consume nutrition as given below:

- Calories needed to gain mass
- You need 18 calories for each pound of the weight of your body
- Calories needed to lose body weight
- You need 12 calories for each pound of your body weight
- Calories needed to maintain your body weight
- You need 15- 16 calories for each pound of your body weight
- You must consume 30 grams or less of carbohydrates per day. The fewer carbohydrates you consume, the quicker you enter ketosis. It is a very important thing to be remembered in Cyclical Ketogenic Diet since you get only 5-6 days for consuming low carbohydrates.
- During the initial three weeks of Cyclical Ketogenic Diet, you can consume 150 grams of protein or 0.9 grams of proteins for each pound of lean mass, whichever is greater. You can set your goals afterwards such as 1- 1.2 grams of proteins for each pound of lean mass.
- For the remaining needs of calories of your body, you can

eat fats.

Beginning your carb-loading

 To push yourself towards the state of anabolism, you can start your state of carb loading 5 hours before you plan to work out. At this time, you can consume 30-50 grams of carbohydrates in addition to fats and proteins to start faster production of enzymes in the liver. An hour or two before your final exercise, you can combine fructose and glucose to replenish liver glycogen. You can add up more carbohydrates if your body needs.

Loading carbohydrates

Most of the times, people consume anything they can lay their hands on when they are in the carb-loading phase. Even though this is quite slapdash, it still gives results. If you want to go by a more scientific method, you need to follow the guidelines. For instance, you can follow these guides:

For the initial 24 hours: 70% of your calorie intake consists of carbohydrates or 4.5 grams for each pound of your lean mass. Then, you can take 15% of fats and 15% of proteins divided evenly. You need to consume foods with higher

Glycemic Index.

For the subsequent 24 hours: You can consume 60% carbohydrates 15% fats, and 25% proteins, or 2.25 grams for each pound of your lean mass. You should consume foods with lower GI.

Using this guide, you can plan your further meals for the week.

How to re-enter ketosis once you complete the carb-up phase

Once your empty your stock of glycogen in your liver, you can easily reach ketosis again. You can follow the steps given below to do it.

For day 1, you must not eat anything past 6 pm.

For day 2, you can perform heavy weight training after you wake up. This has to be done on empty stomach. Begin your Ketogenic diet with carbohydrates intake of only 0-2%.

When you wake up on the third day, you can perform weight training with medium intensity on empty stomach. You can come back to your regular Ketogenic diet and consume 3-5% carbohydrates.

You can build your Cyclical Ketogenic Diet plan based on the above plan.

The more time you spend on Ketogenic diet, the better your body will adapt for it. If you follow this diet for a year, you can enter ketosis more easily than a person who has just started following Cyclical Ketogenic Diet for a month.

More training gives you more scope for entering ketosis easily. You can deplete your stores of glycogen easily. Conditioning and resistance gives you better outcomes than you have with aerobic training. Moreover, if you make wise choices for carb-intake, i.e. foods that have lower GI; you will find it easier to enter ketosis.

You have to remain consistent with the Cyclical Ketogenic Diet to make it easier to re-enter ketosis. If you do not cheat and perform carb-ups properly, your body will adapt to ketosis more easily.

How much intensity is too high for the body?

Normally, anaerobic exercises that occur at repeated intervals and use ruptures of strength can be considered workouts with high intensity.

Workouts with high intensity

- Low repetitions when you do weights above 80% of one repetition at the max.
- Circuit training
- Wrestling or sprinting

Workouts with low intensity

- High repetitions when you do weights above 80% of one repetition at the max.
- Marathon running or jogging
- Yoga

You must not use Cyclical Ketogenic Diet to enhance your limit of endurance. Instead, you can use it to help you conquer the barriers of strength.

Restricted Ketogenic Diet (Therapeutic Uses)

Ketogenic diet can also be used for therapeutic purposes and even conditions like cancer can be cured with Keto. When you confine your carbohydrates intake to 30-50 grams, the body starts depleting its stores of glycogen and begins generating ketone bodies. The healthy cells of your body can utilize ketones for creating energy, but not the cancer cells. The cancer cells are forced to die with this process because glucose is the primary food the cancer causing cells. Studies have actually proven that tumor cells in the pancreas use fructose to divide and reproduce.

When you combine Ketogenic diet with calorie constraint, the body efficiently becomes hostile to the cancer cells. According to some doctors, you can fast on water for the initial 3-5 days. Then, you can start consuming Ketogenic diet with low calories, and aim for the 55-65 mg/ dL of blood sugar and 4 m.M level of blood ketones. It means that you cannot consume more than 20 grams of net carbohydrates per day.

Other than cancer, Ketogenic diet is also used to treat conditions like neurological diseases such as Parkinson's disease, Alzheimer's disease, autism, migraines, depression, and epilepsy; polycystic ovarian syndrome; chronic fatigue syndrome, and many more.

You must note that you must not start therapeutic uses of Ketogenic diet on your own. You must do any kind of dietary experiments under expert medical supervision, especially if you are already taking any medications.

Which kind of Ketogenic diet you should follow?

After reading all kinds of Ketogenic diets, you might be feeling fascinated towards Cyclical Ketogenic Diet or Targeted Ketogenic Diet. However, as said already, only Standard Ketogenic Diet is meant for most people. It is a better option for people who do not indulge in much physical activity.

You can describe Ketogenic diet in fewest words as: low carb, real food, and weight loss. Many of the Ketogenic foods are Paleo friendly as well. It is also important to know that all of the low-carb foods are not healthy. For instance, foods from Atkins diet are full of additives and may cause your insulin level to shoot up. They often contain wheat gluten in pasta alternatives or low-carb breads, which is a crime to eat for a Keto follower. You must choose your foods carefully if you want to achieve your goals.

CHAPTER 2

Important warnings and precautions when using the Ketogenic Diet

The side effects of low- carb diets can be managed if you understand their causes and cures. Once you recognize the physical reactions of your body, you can prevent the worse symptoms of Ketogenic diet and keep you away from quitting too soon. When you adapt to your new diet, you can subside these side effects. You can read the most common side effects on kids and adults that are given below and the methods to cure them.

The adverse effects of Ketogenic diet are less severe than the side effects of anticonvulsant medicines that are used to cure epilepsy. Still, many individuals who follow Ketogenic diet experience several undesirable effects.

Side effects in short term

When you begin the Ketogenic diet, you might experience

several short term effects, especially when you begin the diet with fasting. Hypoglycemia can be commonly observed in this case, which displays these symptoms:

- Frequent urination

- Excessive thirst

- Hunger

- Fatigue

- Confusion, irritability, or anxiety

- Tachycardia

- Shakiness and light headedness

- Chills and sweating

People new to ketosis may also endure low- grade acidosis and constipation. When you continue the diet, you may improve these effects since the body acclimatizes to the new regime and amends the ways it creates energy.

Alternation in the composition of blood

Since the dietary composition changes, the body has to adapt the mechanism to deal with the excessively low consumption of carbohydrates. Additionally, the composition of blood also changes in the Ketogenic diet. The level of cholesterol and lipids in the blood become higher than normal. Over 60% people following Ketogenic diet observe increased level of lipids and 30% people following the new regime observe increased cholesterol level. In case the changes are intense and they seriously affect the health of a person, the diet can be slightly changed. For instance, you can substitute the saturated fats for their polyunsaturated counterparts. You can even lower the ratio of Ketogenic foods and reduce the amount of fats in comparison to proteins and carbohydrates.

Effects in the long term

While you plan to adapt the Ketogenic diet for the long term, you must get frequent health check-ups from a certified medical practitioner. This is because there are a few long term effects of Ketogenic diet that occur in some individuals and they must be treated in time.

Nephrolithiasis or kidney stones are commonly observed in kids following Ketogenic diet. However, kidney stone is easily curable and you can comfortably continue the Ketogenic diet. Hypercalciuria or hypocitraturia are believed to be the causes of kidney stones, when acidosis causes demineralization of bones. Moreover, the low level of pH in the urine promotes the formation of little crystals that result in kidney stones.

There is evidence that when potassium citrate is supplemented, it lowers the chances of stones in kidney since it binds to calcium and lowers the calcium level in the stream of blood. However, more research has to be done in this area.

Children sticking to Ketogenic diet may be influenced by impeded growth because the lower insulin levels. These hormones have an important role in the development of kids, which may get reduced because of Ketogenic diet. Another important long term risk of Ketogenic diet is bone fractures. It arises because of lower insulin level and outcome of acidosis. Bones are eroded because of acidosis and they become weak, which makes them susceptible to fractures.

For people who follow Ketogenic diet, the medical practitioners often prescribe supplements of minerals and vitamins such as vitamin D, calcium, and multivitamin supplements.

Side effects for adults

Adults following Ketogenic diet often see symptoms such as constipation, weight loss, and enhanced levels of triglycerides and cholesterols. Women may experience disruptions in the menstrual cycle and amenorrhea.

Frequent Urination

You might find yourself urinating more often than normal on your first day of Ketogenic diet. This is because your body burns extra glycogen stored in the muscles and livers, which requires significant amount of water. Moreover, when the level of insulin drops, the kidneys excrete sodium causing more urination.

Dizziness and Fatigue

Since you urinate a lot in Ketogenic diet, your body loses minerals like magnesium, potassium, and salt; which can make you feel the fatigue and dizziness. You can keep sipping some salty broth all through the day, or eat foods rich in potassium. You must keep high blood pressure in check in case you have this condition.

Headaches

When your body adapts to ketosis, you may observe frequent headaches for a few days because of mineral loss. You can check it by drinking salt water; if you feel better in 20 minutes, it is because of loss of minerals. You will feel better in 3-4 days.

Constipation

Constipation is a common side effect of Ketogenic diet, which happens because of eating excess of nuts, dehydration, or magnesium potassium imbalance.

Sugar Cravings

Since your body is in the process of burning fats in place of sugar, you might feel intense sugar or carbohydrates cravings during the first 2-3 weeks. These cravings will disappear or subside if you do nit cheat.

Diarrhea

This is also a common side effect of this diet, which will disappear in a few days. It happens because of low intake of fat and high intake of fats and proteins. You can overcome dehydration by eating saturated fat like coconut oil or butter, fattier cut if animal meat, eat heavy cream, etc.

Weakness or Shakiness

Low blood sugar and lower amount of minerals causes shakiness or weakness. You can add more proteins and salt in your foods to counterbalance the dropping of blood sugar.

Muscle Cramps

If you feel cramps in your muscles, you can take tablets of magnesium, but you must talk to your doctor if you have problems in your kidney.

Sleep Disturbances

Many people face problem sleeping when they start following the Ketogenic diet because of low serotonin and insulin levels. When you go to sleep, you can try eating snacks containing carbohydrates and proteins.

A racing heart of heart palpitations

You might experience a racing heart for a few weeks of starting the Ketogenic diet, particularly if you often experience low blood pressure.

CHAPTER 3

Types of Fats in Ketogenic Diet

You might have heard about three kinds of fats in your daily life. However, much misinformation and misconceptions about fats have created over time. Almost all fat types are healthy and important for our body. You must incorporate them in your diet. There is a dominant fat in the food that we eat. For instance, olive oil contains 75% monounsaturated fat and butter contains 60% saturated fats

When you are on a Ketogenic diet, it is particularly important for you to eat the right kind of fats since 70% of your calorie intake comes from fats. Before you read about fats in detail, here is the summary of kinds of fats for you to remember easily.

Good quality Fats

Saturated Fats: Saturated Fats are found in butter, red meat, ghee, cream, lard, eggs, and palm oil/ coconut oil (MCTs).

Monounsaturated Fats: Monounsaturated Fats are found in avocados, extra virgin olive oil, macadamia nut oil, and avocado oil.

Natural Trans Fats: Natural Trans Fats are found in dairy products and meat of grass fed animals.

Natural Polyunsaturated Fats: Natural Polyunsaturated Fats are found in fish oil, fish, chia seeds, and flaxseed.

Even though seeds and legumes are not prohibited in Ketogenic diet, you must eat them in moderation since they contain high amount of Omega-6. You must consume Omega-3 and Omega-6 in almost equal ratio.

Bad Quality Fats

Processed Polyunsaturated Fats: Processed Polyunsaturated Fats are not good for health for Ketogenic followers. They are found in seed oils and vegetables such as Canola, Sesame, Soybean, Corn, Grapeseed, Sunflower, and Peanut.

Processed Trans Fats: Processed Trans Fats are found in margarine, commercially baked foods, and processed foods.

Most of the food you consume in Ketogenic regime should contain monounsaturated and saturated fats. Now, let us study about these fats in detail.

Saturated Fatty Acids

Saturated fats are important to keep the immune system in good health and maintain bone density and testosterone at normal level. Saturated fats were wrongly considered unhealthy for a long time, but recent studies have proved their benefits for the body. In addition, as opposed to the popular myth, they are not bad for your heart. They can be found in Butter, Red meat, Ghee, Eggs, Lard, Cream, Coconut oil (MCTs), Palm oil, Cocoa Butter- just simple foods that have been the part of our diet since ages. They are responsible for improving LDL/ HDL cholesterol level.

Saturated fats enhance the concentration of LDL, which is good for you since cholesterol is important for the body. It is utilized for the creation of hormones such as cortisol and testosterone, which are vital for our good health.

LDL or Low Density Lipoprotein serves the purpose of transportation for cholesterol. Cholesterol moves around the body with the help of LDL. LDL is present in the body in four sizes:

(Dense LDL) very small LDL/ small LDL: These LDL is very small and they can easily seep in through the arterial wall. They are also responsible for causing premature disease of coronary artery.

Intermediate LDL or large LDL: These LDL are large and they are not linked with the enhanced danger of heart ailments.

When you consume good quantities of saturated fat, large LDL increases in the blood and small LDL decreases.

Saturated fats increased the amount of HDL or High Density Lipoprotein. HDL takes out the cholesterol from the blood. It averts build up in arteries because of very small and small LDL. They improve the ratio of LDL and HDL, which must be close to 1:1.

Monounsaturated Fatty Acids or MUFAs

Monounsaturated Fatty Acids also come in the category of healthy fats. They improve your resistance for insulin and enhance the ratio of HDL and LDL. Sunflower and olive oil are the main source of monounsaturated fats. They stabilize blood pressure, protect photo ageing of skin, increase HDL, and cut down belly fat. MUFAs are found in Avocados, Extra virgin olive oil, Macadamia nut oil, Avocado oil, Lard, Bacon fat, and Goose Fat.

Processed Polyunsaturated Fatty Acids (PUFAs)

Polyunsaturated Fatty Acids are usually found in vegetable oils. They are typically highly processed, but you should stay away from so-called heart healthy vegetable oils such as corn, soybean, sunflower, and canola oils. These oils go through tremendous processing that involve several solvents, chemicals, bleach, and many more harmful things. They are also high in Omega-6 fatty acids. Recent studies have shown that liquid Trans fats and vegetable oils are responsible for heart diseases, not the saturated fats. They worsen the LDL/ HDL level.

Natural Polyunsaturated Fatty Acids

On the other hand, natural sources of polyunsaturated fats are good for you such as fatty fish, flaxseed, fish oil, Chia seeds, etc. They improve the level of LDL/ HDL cholesterol and contain high concentration of Omega-3 fatty acids. You must consume more foods containing natural PUFAs. As told above, you must maintain the ratio of 1:1 for Omega-6 and Omega-3.

Trans Fatty Acids

Although Trans fats are not incorporated in fatty foods, they need special mention. They are made from unnatural chemical processes that give them more shelf life. Hydrogenation is one of the processes, which includes adding hydrogen to Trans Fatty Acids. It alters the placement of hydrogen atoms inside the chain of fatty acids. In the nutshell, whenever you see the label of a food packet with the words 'hydrogenated' or 'trans fats', you must not eat it. Trans Fatty Acids are terrible for your health and disrupt your level of LDL/HDL cholesterol.

TFAs are the unhealthiest form of fats available in the market. Hydrogenation involved securing polyunsaturated oils so that they do not become rancid. Hydrogenated fats are utilized in fast foods, processed foods, commercially baked foods, and margarine. You must stay away from such foods when you are making so much effort for your Ketogenic diet. Processed TFAs are the common cause of coronary heart diseases. They are also linked with numerous long standing problems related to health such as breast cancer, depression, and obesity.

Natural Trans Fatty Acids

Natural TFAs are found in grass fed animal and dairy fat. Grain-fed animals do not contain much of natural TFAs. They are healthy for human body and protect us against cancer, helps lose body fat, lowers hypertension, and provides several other biological benefits.

It is essential to eat high amount of fat in Ketogenic diets, but you have to make sure that you take the right type of fat. You must know the right temperature of cooking for various oils. Avocado oil and olive oil are best implemented for cold use or light cooking. Ghee, butter, coconut oil, and bacon fat are best used for cooking on high heat.

Fat and cholesterol

Cholesterol constantly moves around in the body. Therefore, it is essential that these particles do not face many crashes in the artery walls because it builds plaque. HDL can be called as good element and LDL can be labeled as bad cholesterol. HDL transfers cholesterol from tissues of the body into the liver for break them down. LDL, on the other hand, picks he processed cholesterol from liver and sends it back to tissues of the body. That is why it is recommended to have a balance 1:1 ratio of LDL and HDL. Fat takes the form of triglycerides when it is carried around in the stream of blood. Although triglycerides do not cause bad cholesterol, they indicate it.

When the LDL count is low in the body, you can afford to have small particles of LDL to carry cholesterol through the stream of blood since they have to avoid less traffic. If you have high count of LDL, the traffic increases in the bloodstream and hence, the possibilities of crashes increase. If you have large particles of LDL and low count of LDL, crashes will hardly occur. Cholesterol can be easily transported through the bloodstream.

We must consider triglycerides since they also move in the bloodstream. They consume extra space, so if you have high count of triglycerides, you will need higher count of LDL particles. If more number of LDL particles are there, probability of crashes increases.

CHAPTER 4

Foods you can eat in Ketogenic Diet

Since you are going to eat lots of fat in Ketogenic diet, you have to make choices based on your digestive tolerance. Most people are not able to digest mayonnaise or vegetable oil, or even Olive oil for a long time. You can refer to the list of foods recommended in this diet and keep away from non-recommended foods as much as you can. It is not possible to remember all the things mentioned in the list. Therefore, you can just keep the concepts of Ketogenic diet in mind and broadly keep the list in mind. If you cannot recall whether you should eat something or not, just try to recall the logics and you will be able to make a wise choice.

Oils and fats

- Avocado
- Avocado oil
- Beef tallow of grass fed cattle
- Almond oil
- Organic Butter

- Organic Chicken fat
- Organic Duck fat
- Ghee
- organic leaf lard
- Macadamia oil
- Macadamia Nuts
- Mayonnaise
- Olives
- Organic Olive oil
- Organic coconut oil,
- Coconut cream concentrate
- Organic Red Palm oil
- Coconut butter
- Peanut Butter
- Seed and nut oils: Flaxseed oil, Sesame oil, etc (do not heat)
- 85-90% dark chocolate

Protein sources

- Grass fed Meat: lamb, beef, veal, goat, or wild game
- Pork: Boston butt, pork loin, ham, pork chops
- Poultry: chicken, quail, turkey, Cornish hen, pheasant, duck, goose

- Fish or any kind of seafood, if possible wild caught: calamari, catfish, anchovies, cod, flounder, herring, mackerel, halibut, mahi-mahi, sardines, salmon, scrod, sole, trout, tuna, and snapper.

- Canned salmon and tuna are good enough but you must check their labels for fillers or added sugars.

- Shellfish: clams, lobster, crab, scallops, shrimp, mussels, squid, and oysters

- Whole eggs: deviled, hard-boiled, fried, omelets, scrambled, soft-boiled, and poached

- Sausage and Bacon: avoid products that contain fillers or sugar like wheat and soy.

- Soy products and Peanut butter such as tofu, edamame, and tempeh have good amount of of protein, but also high amount of carbohydrates, so eat them wisely.

- Whey protein powders, and pea, rice, hemp and or other powders of vegetable protein. Whey protein spikes insulin, so eat them carefully.

Fresh Vegetables

Most of the non-starchy vegetables do not contain many

carbohydrates. You must buy organic vegetables. If you do not get organic variants, you can try growing them on your own so that there is no chance of pesticide residues. Avoid vegetables containing starch such as peas, corn, sweet potatoes, potatoes, and winter squash. Limit consumption of sweeter vegetables like carrots, tomatoes, summer squashes, and peppers.

- Alfalfa Sprouts
- Asparagus
- Leafy green vegetable
- Avocado
- Bean Sprouts
- Bamboo Shoots
- Beet Greens
- Bok choy
- Bell peppers*
- Broccoli
- Cabbage
- Brussels sprouts
- Carrots*
- Celery
- Cauliflower
- Chard

- Celery root
- Chives
- Cucumbers
- Collard greens
- Dandelion greens
- Garlic
- Dill pickles
- Kale
- Salad greens and Lettuces (Boston lettuce, arugula, chicory, escarole, endive, fennel, mache, romaine, radicchio, sorrel)
- Leeks
- Mushrooms
- Olives
- Radishes
- Onions*
- Sauerkraut (watch for added sugar)
- Shallots
- Scallions
- Snow Peas
- Sprouts
- Spinach
- Summer squash*

- Swiss chard
- Turnips
- Tomatoes*

* Eat these vegetables in moderation.

Dairy Products

You can consume raw milk products. Some of the dairy products trigger insulin. Therefore, it is better to limit their quantity of consumption.

- Heavy whipped cream
- Cottage cheese (full fat)
- Sour cream (full fat)
- All soft and hard cheeses- one ounce contains almost 1 carb
- Cream cheese
- Whole milk yogurt (unsweetened)
- Mascarpone cheese

Seeds and Nuts

Soak and roast the seeds and nuts to remove their anti-nutrients. They contain high amount of carbohydrates and calories. Therefore, eat them in moderation.

- Nuts: pecans, macadamias, walnuts, and almonds have lowest amount of carbohydrates. Pistachios, cashews, and chestnuts contain high amount of carbohydrates, so track them carefully.
- Nut flours like almond flour.
- Peanuts in limited amount
- Seeds of pumpkin, sesame, sunflower, etc..

Beverages

- Bone broth, Clear broth
- Decaf coffee
- Unsweetened decaf tea
- Unsweetened herbal tea
- Water
- Unsweetened flavored seltzer water
- Lemon and lime juice
- Unsweetened almond milk
- Unsweetened coconut milk
- Unsweetened soy milk

Sweeteners

If you can avoid sweetened foods completely, you can reset your taste buds. However, if you still want to eat something sweet, you can eat anything from the list given below. You must know that the powdered sweeteners usually contain dextrose, maltodextrin, or any other kind of sugar. Therefore, you must prefer liquid sweeteners.

- Liquid Stevia
- Erythritol
- Xylitol (food containint xylitol must be kept at distance from dogs.
- Liquid Splenda*
- Monk Fruit
- Lo Han Guo
- Chicory Root and Inulin

Splenda is a controversial sweetener, but research has been done to prove that it can be consumed by Ketogenic followers.

Fruits and other miscellaneous foods

- Berries (strawberries, raspberries, blueberries) can be eaten occasionally in limited portions.
- Pork Rinds

- Japanese Shirataki noodles

Spices

Spices also contain carbohydrates, so count the calories before you add them to your meals. Commercial mixes of spices contain added sugar. You can use sea salt in place if commercial salt, which contains powdered dextrose.

- Ground allspice
- Dried basil
- Black pepper
- Ground cardamom
- Caraway seed
- Cayenne pepper
- Ground cinnamon
- Coriander seeds
- Cloves
- Curry powder
- Garlic powder
- Fennel seeds
- Ground ginger
- Vanilla extract
- Ground mace

- Nutmeg
- Ground oregano
- Onion powder
- Paprika
- Dried parsley
- Fresh peppermint
- Poultry seasoning
- Poppy seeds
- Pumpkin pie spice
- Ground sage
- Dried spearmint
- Ground tarragon
- Ground thyme
- White pepper
- Vanilla extract

Foods you must avoid in Ketogenic diet

- All grains, white potatoes and quinoa
- Whole meal grains- rye, oats, wheat, corn, barley, bulgur, sorghum, millet, rice, amaranth, sprouted grains, buckwheat
- Products made from grains- bread, pasta, pizza, crackers, cookies

- Sweets and sugar- HFCS, table sugar, ice creams, agave syrup, cakes, soft-drinks, sweet puddings
- Factory farmed fish and pork
- Processed foods, MSG products, BPAs, sulphites
- Artificial sweeteners- Splenda, Equal, and sweeteners containing Acesulfame, Aspartame, Saccharin, Sucralose, etc
- Refined oils/ fats- safflower, sunflower, cottonseed, soybean, canola, corn oil grapeseed; and Trans fats like margarine
- Zero carb, low carb, low fat products
- High amount of milk is not recommended. You can take it in limited quantity
- Sweet drinks and alcoholic drinks- sweet wine, beer, cocktails, etc.
- Tropical fruits- pineapple, papaya, mango, banana
- Fruits high in carbohydrates- grapes, tangerine
- Fruit juices including fresh juices (you can take smoothies if you want)
- Soy products
- Wheat gluten
- Cans lined with BPA
- Carrageenan
- Sulfites in gelatin, dried fruits

CONCLUSION

For those who do not know much about Ketogenic diet may get too excited about the results this regime gives, and that too without exercising vigorously. And now that you have read so much about Ketogenic diet, you are aware of its pros and cons. So you must know how you can manage your body before you begin a new regime.

Ketogenic diet has beautiful effects if you want to have a lean body without making much effort in exercising. And if you are a person who loves working out vigorously, there are other sub-divisions of Ketogenic diet such as Cyclical Ketogenic Diet or Target Ketogenic Diet. The latter options give you the choice of eating carbohydrates, but must not take it as an excuse to eat carbohydrates. This is allowed only because the diet demands so.

It is easy for adults to start this diet since they can handle the side effects of Keto quite well, but you can also make your children adapt to this diet. Children have more capability to adapt to new things, but you must keep them under professional medical supervision since they are prone to permanent side effects of Ketogenic diet. We have to make sure that they receive appropriate amount of minerals that our body loses when the insulin level becomes very low.

In case you are a patient of high/ low blood pressure, diabetes, or any other medical condition, you must consult your doctor before you begin Ketogenic diet. This diet gives amazing results in terms of weight loss and health effects in the long term, but you have to abide by its rules. If you do not lose hope in the first few weeks, your body will surely adapt to Ketogenic diet and your will soon witness the results.